INTERMITTENT FASTING

Simple Guide to Weight Loss, Fat Loss and Improved Health

The Fat Loss and Anti Aging Diet

VALERIE CHILDS

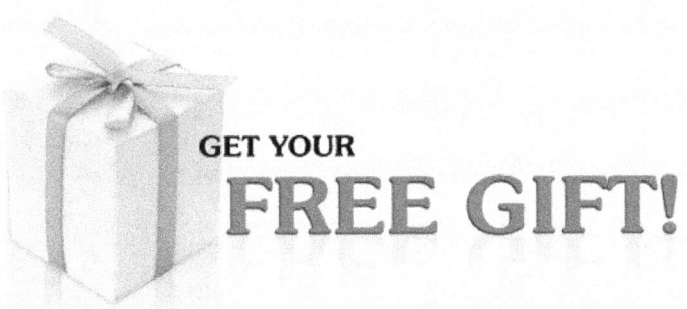

GET YOUR

FREE GIFT!

WAIT! – DO YOU LIKE FREE BOOKS?

My FREE Gift to You!! As a way to say Thank You for downloading my book, I'd like to offer you more FREE BOOKS! Each time we release a NEW book, we offer it first to a small number of people as a test - drive. Because of your commitment here in downloading my book, I'd love for you to be a part of this group. You can join easily here → **http://www.fatlosswithpaleo.com**

TABLE OF CONTENTS

INTRO

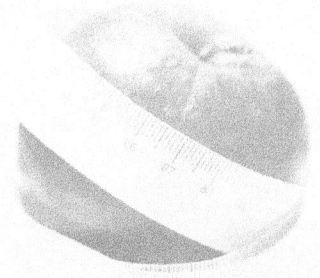

We live in an era where lifestyle diseases have become bigger health threats than diseases that were once and still are feared. Heart disease is currently the top killer in the United States, claiming around 600,000 lives every year. It is also the leading cause of deaths in most other parts of the world.

Obesity currently affects 34.9% of adults in the United States. Thats around 78 million people, more than a third of the entire population.

The bad news is that things are not getting better. The statistics are growing worse with every year. One of the main causes of this worsening situation is a high level of misinformation available today, especially on websites and from so called experts. People are following fad diets and ineffective, usually dangerous, weight loss methods.

CHAPTER 1

WHAT IS INTERMITTENT FASTING?

But there is one weight loss method that if done right, will help you lose weight and improve your health. This is intermittent fasting. It is a dieting plan that involves alternating a period of eating with a period of restricted or no eating at all. Numerous studies have backed up the fact that intermittent fasting is highly beneficial in weight loss and overall body health.

In this book you will learn the types of intermittent fasting, common myths surrounding the practice, benefits of intermittent fasting and how to do it yourself.

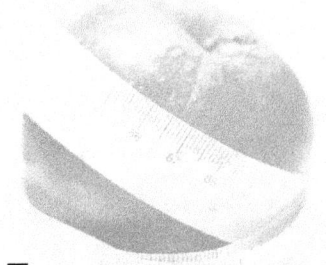

CHAPTER 2

THE 5 TOP INTERMITTENT FASTING METHODS

There are different approaches to fasting. Read through them and see which one fits best into your life and situation. Whichever you choose, the most important thing is to have a fast that lasts between 12-24 hours for scientific reasons to be explained shortly. You can choose how long to carry out the fast between these hours.

1. Eat Stop Eat method

This method advocates for a full 24 hours of fasting once or twice a week. During the fast, it is recommended that you drink calorie-free beverages to keep your body well hydrated. This is one of the most popular intermittent fasting methods.

It is loved mostly because of its simplicity. All you have to do is select one or two days in a week when you will fast. In addition to its freeing simplicity, it has also been reported to be highly effective in weight loss. It also comes with many other health benefits.

2. Leangains method

Martin Berkhan has a highly recommended method that has led to tons of success stories. He, after rigorous research, recommends a 14 hours of fasting for women and 16 for men. This means that men have a feeding period of 8 hours while that of women is 10 hours.

The method is simple and easy to follow with clear guidelines. The best part about it is its easy adaptation into someone's life. Martin has different protocols for trainers, students and for those with normal working hours.

Compared to most other types of intermittent fasting, Leangains is the easiest to adopt into a lifestyle. It however requires getting used to the somewhat tight food restrictions during the fast period.

3. The Warrior Diet

In the strictest of terms, this is not an intermittent fasting method. Rather, it is a partial daily fast with a 20/4 fast/feed routine. This means fasting for 20 hours and feeding for the remaining 4 hours in a day. The reason why we refer to it as a partial diet is because it allows small meals such as fruits and vegetables during the 20 hour fast.

It can be a major challenge to turn the Warrior Diet into a lifestyle considering that for most part of the day, it does not allow large meals. This makes a social life very difficult and sometimes awkward.

Generally, this technique works best for people who are looking for a quick way to lose weight.

4. Feast/Fast method

This technique is a bit unusual in that it allows for a full day of cheating. You can eat whatever you desire. After this, you go on a 36 hour fast.

This method has several downsides. For one, it is easy to binge on unhealthy foods during the cheat day, especially after 36 hours of fasting. Secondly, most people may not be used to fasting for 36 hours and may therefore be unable to do it.

5. Alternate Day Diet

Like its name suggests, this method involves alternating your fasting days. On one day you eat normally with the usual calorie intake. On fasting days, rather than going without any food, you restrict your diet to 20% of the normal calorie intake. This means taking in around 400 to 500 calories.

Like the warrior approach, the Alternate day Diet is very friendly towards weight loss. But it is a bit harder to adopt it as a nutritional lifestyle.

CHAPTER 3

WHICH ONE IS BEST FOR YOU?

The answer to this question is highly subjective. There is no one method that is perfect for everyone. each technique has its own goals and expectations. Before you make a choice, ask yourself several questions:

What are my goals?
Do I want something permanent or temporary?
How is my social life?
How is my work and training schedule?

Choose a method that helps you reach your objective e.g a healthier lifestyle or quick weight loss and fits well into your day without causing any complications.

CHAPTER 4

DEBUNKING THE TOP 10 MOST COMMON WEIGHT LOSS AND NUTRITION MYTHS

D espite all the benefits it has to offer (which will be discussed later) intermittent fasting has received a lot of bad rap from people who don't want to examine proven facts. For this reason, a number of myths about the practice have been spread around.

1. Eating 6 Small Meals a Day Boosts Metabolism and Helps in Weight Loss! (FALSE)

This is one of the most common myths around. Its supporters recommend ditching the three square meals a day routine, for six small meals in a day. The stated benefits include higher metabolism and faster weight loss.

There is however, no proven truth in the above. In fact, it is scientifically impossible to enjoy those benefits by following the 5-6 small meals a day routine. A number of research studies have seen no connection between higher meal frequency and weight loss or better health.

The most important thing to understand is this, the number of calories your body burns throughout the day is not dependent on meal frequency. In weight loss, what matters most is the difference between the number of calories taken in and those used up by the body. Regardless of your meal frequency, you will gain weight if at the end of the day, you eat more calories than you expend.

2. Breakfast is the Most Important Meal for Weight Loss! (FALSE)

This is another common one that has been tossed around for so long that so many people believe it. Breakfast is commonly referred to as the most important meal for the day. Thanks to recent research however, this has been disproven. Being a loyal breakfast eater will not help you lose weight just as missing it will not lead to weight gain.

The thinking is that missing breakfast leaves one hungry. It becomes easier therefore, to snack and overeat during the day. But various rigorous studies have seen no major differences in the amount of weight lost between breakfast eaters and skippers.

What matters is not whether you eat breakfast or not but what you eat.

3. Intermittent Fasting Will Make You Lose Muscle! (FALSE)

One of the scare tactics used to keep people from experiencing the benefits of proper fasting is saying that it causes loss of muscle tissue. While you certainly want fat to burn away, hearing that your muscle will go to will cause some hesitation.

But the root of this myth is a misunderstanding of the body's protein intake process. Proteins are the sources of amino acids that keep muscles healthy and growing. Once you eat a meal containing proteins, that is enough to produce amino acids for more than 16 hours.

As you will see later, this book book recommends a fasting period of between 12-24 hours. You are therefore in no danger of muscle tissue depletion.

You only lose muscle tissue in cases of extreme starvation. If the glycogen, a source of energy, stored in the liver runs out, the body turns to muscle tissue for energy.

4. Do Not Workout During Fast! (FALSE)

This myth suggests that fasted training is bad for you because you will lose muscle and have no strength. But it is interesting to note that studies have shown that even three days of fasting do not affect training performance. So for intermittent fasting that only lasts for a few hours, you have nothing to worry about.

To make your training highly effective however, it is recommended that you take a pre and post workout protein supplement. Some BCAA powder or tablets are the best.

5. Eating at Night Will Cause Weight Gain! (FALSE)

A common saying that you should start your day with a King's breakfast and end it with a Pauper's dinner. There is a misconception that the more you eat at night the higher the possibility of weight gain. The belief is that when asleep, the body burns a lot less calories and the unused calories are turned into fat.

Again, calories in versus calories out is what matters. As long as you are not snacking on unhealthy, high calorie junk food or overeating, you should be okay. In fact, one study connected people who ate large evening meals with more muscle growth. You therefore don't need to starve yourself in the evening simply because of the fear of weight gain.

6. Eat Smaller Meals Throughout the Day Controls Hunger! (FALSE)

The myth of more smaller meals is not only confined to metabolism, its proponents also add hunger control as one of its benefits. The (wrong) recommendation is that, instead of there large meals during the course of the entire day, you should have six small ones. This ensures that you do not feel hungry and as a result, you will not overeat or get tempted to snack unhealthily.

Science has once again come to the rescue. Several studies have shown no evidence of the above being true. In fact, research leans more towards the three square meals a day plan. Eating three large meals, instead of six smaller ones, results in much better appetite control.

7. Eating Smaller Meals Controls Blood Sugar! (FALSE)

This is another of the many smaller meals myths. First it was to maintain metabolism and high energy levels throughout the day. Then it was to control hunger. Now, it is to control blood sugar levels.

What many people don't understand is that the human body is extremely good at keeping blood sugar levels in check. Whether you fats for 12 hours, 36 hours or three days, your blood sugar will remain the same. This exception was most probably carried over from our ancestors through evolution.

8. Fasting Forces the Body into a Destructive Starvation Mode! (FALSE)

Starvation refers to an extreme body state where metabolic rate slows down drastically and energy level fall. At this point, the body is doing its best to stay alive for as long as possible. Now, do you think that a few hours of fasting will get you here? Certainly not.

A lot of studies have collaborated the view that starvation can take up to 96 hours before it occurs. The first drop in resting metabolic rate happens after around 60 hours of fasting. Most interesting is the fact that in the short term (up to 60 hours) the metabolic rate actually ruses. The explanation for this is related to the lifestyle of our pre-evolutionary ancestors.

This rise in metabolic rate is what causes a boost of energy and a sharper mental focus for people undertaking intermittent fasting.

9. Eating Protein every 2-3 Hours per Day is Needed to Support Muscle Growth! (FALSE)

Athletes and trainers are frequently advised to eat a diet choke full of proteins. Even worse is the suggestion that they should eat a high protein meal every 2 to 3 hours. This, supposedly ensures the steady flow of amino acids to the muscles thus ensuring effective workouts. The myth is further fueled by the claims that the body can only take in 30 grams of proteins during a meal, thus the justification for the frequent protein fixes.

The truth is that you can have amino acids trickling into your bloodstream hours after finishing a high protein meal. You do not need to keep bombarding the body with additional proteins. In fact, experts say that a normal meal contains enough proteins for athletes and trainers.

10. Fasting Increases Stress Levels Due to Abnormal Releases of Cortisol! (FALSE)

Normal release of the hormone cortisol is very important for a number of reasons. It helps regulate the circadian rhythm, arousing us in the morning. It is the hormone responsible for giving you an elevated mood important for starting the day well. It is also necessary in the function of the immune system and blood pressure maintenance.

If too much of it is released, stress levels shoot up. In some cases it can lead to serious depression. This is the fact that has been distorted to make fasting look like a bad thing. Fasting does not increase cortisol levels in the body and scientific research supports this position.

CHAPTER 5

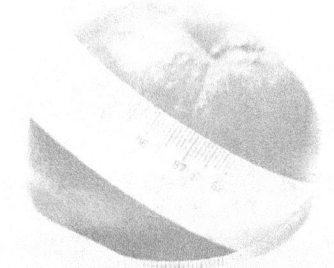

INTERMITTENT FASTING AND WEIGHT LOSS

For a lot of people interested in learning more about intermittent fasting, they are doing it so as to lose weight and become lean (less fat, more muscle). If you are such a person then good news is, yes, you can lose weight through intermittent fasting. It is not magic bullet or a shortcut to weight loss. You still need to have discipline, determination, willpower and most importantly patience.

If you really want to succeed in losing weight through intermittent fasting, you need to be ready to adopt it as a lifestyle, not a diet. This is not a three day crash diet to get you slim, it is a lifestyle that takes weeks to give you great results.

CHAPTER 6

THE SCIENCE BEHIND INTERMITTENT FASTING WEIGHT LOSS

One thing that should make you feel good about taking up this lifestyle is all the scientific support it has. It is not something dreamed up by a diet guru'. Solid research and evidence supports its adoption.

The science behind intermittent fasting weight loss is mostly about how the body produces its energy. When you eat, sugar is stored in the liver in form of glycogen. The body uses it to produce energy. When you eat a meal during breakfast, lunch and dinner, your body will never run out of glycogen to use for energy synthesis. There is therefore no time when it will turn to fat burning for energy.

The only problem is, you want your body to burn fat so as to reduce it and lose weight. The only way to do this is wait until glycogen is depleted, then force the body to burn fat. Intermittent fasting does this.

It takes about 8-12 hours, without further eating, for glycogen to run out. This is why it is recommended that any intermittent fasting method should not run for less than 12 hours. After 8-12 hours, the body turns to fat for its energy needs. To help in burning more fat, you can engage in exercises such as cardio workouts or weight lifting.

With continued adherence to intermittent fasting, you can get to a point where the body adapts to using fat more than glycogen. At this time, maintaining a healthy body weight is far much easier. For some people the process can take a few weeks while for others it can take months. Patience is therefore key.

While a lot regarding intermittent fasting and weight loss has been uncovered through science, a lot more remains to be explained. Researchers continue to dig and so far, the news regarding this nutritional lifestyle is promising. There are tons of studies you can read up on to deepen your knowledge in intermittent fasting and verify the facts presented here.

CHAPTER 7

THE TOP 8 BENEFITS OF INTERMITTENT FASTING

As has been mentioned several times, one of the biggest benefits of intermittent fasting is weight loss. It has been described as a safe and highly effective way to shed the excess pounds and maintain a healthy weight. Even better, its benefits for weight loss are supported by science.

It is important to note that to lose weight through intermittent fasting, it is necessary to adopt it as a lifestyle rather than a temporary diet plan. Only this way can you give it enough time to have the desired effect on the body.

But acceleration of fat loss is not the only impact intermittent fasting is has on the body. Here are several more amazing benefits of this nutritional lifestyle.

1. Improved Mental Focus

Our ancestors who lived in the wild, did not always get something to eat. At times they would go hungry. During such periods of hunger, as an adaptation, mental focus and clarity greatly improved. This helped in better hunting for prey. The same can be observed in wild animals today.

A less extreme version of that happens when you go on a fast. During those hours, your mental focus increases. Completing tasks becomes easier, you are not easily distracted and creativity actually heightens. Essentially your productivity peaks. This is one of the reasons why experts recommend people to undertake their fasting hours during busy times. Not only does it help reduce thoughts on food and hunger, it also takes advantage of the improved mental state.

Beware of the common misconception that eating often keeps the brain sharp. You will hear people telling you that it is important to have an energy bar or protein shake every now and then to stay alert. This is bad because it makes the body dependent on carbs to produce energy. Instead, you should teach it to use fat to power the body and keep the brain sharp.

2. Boosting of Brain Health

Experiments on animals have already shown that intermittent fasting can prevent or prolong the onset of neurological disorders. Early research is uncovering similar benefits in humans. A certain scientific article compared fasting to exercise. In the same way that muscles become stronger through exercise, fasting strengthens the brain.

It accomplishes this through the production of certain chemicals. These chemicals influence brain activity making you more mentally focused, elevating your moods and making your brain healthier.

One specific chemical that has been thoroughly researched is a protein referred to as brain-derived neurotrophic factor or BDNF. This brain boosting protein has been shown to increase in levels during calorie restriction or fasting. The increase can be between 50 and 400 percent. This increase varies depending on the brain region.

What does BDNF do?

- It triggers brain cells to form new neurons thus rejuvenating the brain.

- It triggers the release of various other chemicals that positively affect neural health.

- It protects neural cells from damage such as that caused by Parkinson's and Alzheimer's.

- It also travels to the muscles to protect neuro-motors from damage. The degradation of neuro motors is partly why muscles waste as old age sets in. BDNF can prevent this from happening too quickly.

3. Increase in Insulin Sensitivity

Insulin resistance is a factor that is behind a lot of the chronic diseases that are affecting millions of people all over the world. Such diseases include diabetes, cancer and heart disease.

A body that relies too much on sugar to produce energy is at a higher risk of insulin resistance. When the body adapts to burning more fat instead of sugar, through intermittent fasting, insulin resistance is greatly reduced. With insuline sensitivity increased, blood sugar is transpoted more easily in the blood.

Another way in which intermittent fasting increases insulin sensitivity is by combating obesity. We have already seen how fasting helps in weight loss. Obesity is a major factor in causing insulin resistance. By combating it, fasting positively impacts insulin sensitivity.

4. Increased Longevity Rate

The association between intermittent fasting and longevity are under heavy scrutiny. Initial experiments in rats resulted in a 15 to 20 percent increase in length of life. Monkeys were also seen to experience more longevity with intermittent fasting. Experts think that the same is possible in humans.

One way in which intermittent fasting is though to increase longevity is by increasing the body's ability to resist disease, stress and aging. In fact, fasting affects the body at the cellular level. Individual cells become more resistance to damage or degeneration. Every part of the body starting from the skin to the muscles and the brain stay younger for longer.

5. Easy to Follow and Maintain Long Term

One of the reasons why a large majority of diets never work is because it is impossible to stick to them. Most require an extreme restriction of calories, something that is not possible to maintain for long. So even if one loses weight, it come barreling back as soon as the diet is ditched.

Intermittent fasting is different in that it is not a diet. As mentioned several times, it is a lifestyle you can opt to adopt into your life. This makes it easier to lose weight and actually keep it off. Once you are used to it, you will be able to fast naturally without much effort.

6. Potential Anti-Cancer Benefits

This is another area of intermittent fasting that is in its early stages of study. There is therefore no conclusive evidence that intermittent fasting can help in cancer treatment. In mice, fasting and calorie restriction were quite effective in fighting cancer cells and there is hope that the results can be replicated in humans.

There is however a bigger ray of hope. Research has shown that undertaking intermittent fasting before cancer treatment can improve chances of being cured and also improves tolerance to chemotherapy.

7. Increased Production of Human Growth Hormone (HGH)

HGH is a very important hormone in the body. With the adoption of an intermittent fasting lifestyle, its levels increase in the body. This results in a number of benefits. They include faster and better muscle repair, improved muscle function, better cell regeneration, faster tissue healing and increased energy levels.

8. Anti-Aging at the Cellular Level

Autophagy is a cell process in which cells recycle wastes, reduce or eliminate wasteful cellular processes and carry out cell repair. All of these are extremely important functions. Autophagy helps in anti aging, reducing the atrophy of muscle tissue and in effective muscle function. Intermittent fasting has been shown to boost autophagy in cells.

Other Benefits

- Lower triglyceride levels. This is espcially important in maintaining heart health.

- Normalizing the levels of the hunger hormone, ghrelin. This helps to achieve better appetite control ensuring that any gains made are not lost.

- Lowering inflammation and protecting cells from free radical damage.

Basically, prolonged intermittent fasting leaves your body fitter and healthier than it has ever been.

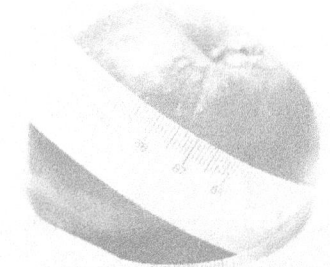

CHAPTER 8

THE 10 STEPS IN STARTING YOUR OWN INTERMITTENT FASTING PROGRAM

You have read a lot of things on intermittent fasting including what it is, they myths surrounding it and most importantly its benefits. Now, we have come to the most important part, applying it in your life. Below is a short guide on how to go about it, important tips to know about and mistakes to avoid.

STEP 1 – Decide on the Best Approach for You

Earlier, we looked at five approaches most commonly used in intermittent fasting. Those approaches suit different people. You should make a decision as to which you will use based on your schedule, objectives and preferences.

If your goal is mainly weight loss for instance, the warrior diet or the feast/fast method are ideal. If you want to build muscle alongside losing weight Marting of Leangains has some pretty great plans that also include recommendation on supplements. If you want an approach that is super simple and very easy to adopt, go for the Eat Stop Eat technique. For an approach with bigger long term benefits go for either Leangains or the Alternate Day diet.

If you are not sure what to choose, you can try several of them. Find an approach that works for you and stick with it.

STEP 2–Start Slowly with Shorter Fasting Periods

A very crucial point to note is that in the beginning, you may not feel all that well about intermittent fasting. This is especially for those who are used to eating a small meal every two hours or so. But you have to be strong and determined. As you continue, your body will adapt into the new lifestyle and it will be much easier.

To help the transition into the new lifestyle, it is advisable that you start slowly and progress from there. Instead of starting with 12 or 20 hours of fasting, let your body get used to 5 hours. You can start by skipping lunch. Alternatively, skip breakfast and eat a small snack before lunch.

As you progress, you should get to a point where the last meal is at 8pm at night and the next full meal at noon the next day.

STEP 3–Plan Your Menu

One common mistake people make is thinking that because they are fasting, they can eat anything they want. To get the full benefits you have to also change your dietary components. Include more fruits and vegetables in your meals and do not forget to drink lots of water. Avoid highly processed foods and high sugar products like Soda and candy.

Having a planned menu before you start ensures that you know what you are going to eat for each meal of the week. Having no plan makes it easy to order an unhealthy meal.

STEP 4–Stay Active

You will feel hungry, expect it. The worst thing you can do when you are hungry is stay idle. You will start thinking about food and soon enough you will give in to the temptations. The best way to spend your fasting hour is by staying busy. Whether you are in the office, your own business or a home project, find something that engages your hands and your mind.

STEP 5–Exercise

To amplify the benefits of intermittent benefit, include regular workouts into your schedule. We have already debunked the myth that fasting makes you weaker and causes a less effective workout. Weight lifting and cardio will help burn even more fat and develop your muscles. Just be careful not to be overzealous with the exercise.

STEP 6–Do Not Overeat or Overdrink

Most types of intermittent fasting allow one to take drinks during the fasting period. Be careful not to take too many drinks that the calories add up quickly. Examples of beverages to avoid too much off include diet soda, coffee and fruit juice.

The same applies to the warrior diet that allows some fruits and veggies. Overeating fruits and some vegetables can lead to a high calorie intake. The word here is moderation.

STEP 7–Do Not Be Afraid of Getting Hungry

When people start out most will dread the prospect of getting hungry. This fear can prevent you from enjoying the benefits of fasting.

Hunger is just a body response that you can learn to cope with. Most importantly, feeling hungry does not mean that you will starve to death or that your muscles will start getting wasted. The body can go for several days without food.

In the beggining it will be difficult to cope with the hunger but you will master it within a short time.

STEP 8–Do Not Starve Yourself

It is normal to think that more of a good thing is better. But this is not the case with intermittent fasting. Simply because fasting for 15 hours has done wonders for you does not mean that 48 hours will too, in fact, it will damage your body.

Prolonged fasting is what is referred to as starvation. Your muscles start to waste, metabolism rate drops and energy levels go down drastically. This kind of fasting is not helpful at all.

Experts recommend the minimum fasting period to be 12 hours and the maximum period to be 20 hours.

STEP 9 – Make it a Habit that Turns into a Lifestyle

If you keep looking at the clock wondering when you can start eating again, you are doing it wrong. try as much as possible to relax while fasting and focus on other things, This is why you should do it when busy. Also, do it until it turns into a habit which then becomes a lifestyle.

STEP 10 – Keep Monitoring Health

Do not fast blindly. Keep checking your health status to ensure that the fasting is not causing any health problems. If you start experiencing serious diziness, fainting or weakness, stop fasting immediately and eat something. It is good to see your doctor to get checked.

CHAPTER 9

THESE PEOPLE SHOULD NOT USE INTERMITTENT FASTING

Since intermittent fasting involves the deprivation of food to the body for hours at a time, there are some people who should not use it lose weight or become healthier. These are people who are at health risks due to fasting. They include:

- Women who are either pregnant or nursing. It is extremely important for babies to receive nutrients for proper growth and development. Fasting for hours can affect the delivery of these nutrients. Furthermore, there is no research that supports the use of intermittent fasting when pregnant or nursing.

- People who are diabetic or hypoglycemic. Such people are at higher health risks. If you have these conditions and want to practice fasting, consult with your doctor first.

Other include people with heart problems, hormonal regulation problems especially cortisol and those experiencing chronic stress. If at all you think fasting might affect you negatively, stay safe and see your doctor before commencing your fast.

Conclusion

Intermittent fasting is not for everyone. As easy as it may seem, others will find it difficult especially if they have to do it over a long period of time. Do not feel pressured to get into a lifestyle that will stress you out. Just eat healthy, do your exercises, lower stress and you will live a long healthy life.

However, you can occassionally try a few hours of fasting for detoxification purposes. It helps your body flush out accumulated toxins and improve in function. If you can manage 12-16 hours of fasting once every week or so, it will benefit you a lot.

For the others who are ready to get into this new lifestyle, all the best. You can do it.

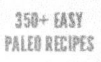 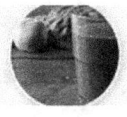 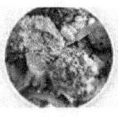 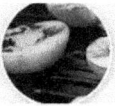 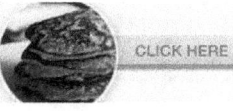

I want to share with you one of my all time favorite Paleo Recipe books! It's literally called, "The Paleo Recipe Book" because really, from what I've seen, this is it. It's all you need. At least until I finish my recipe book. My hope is you at least check it out and try. Please update me on what you think of it.

PLUS I believe you also get extra bonuses to go along with it like a 8 week meal plan, cheat sheets, etc.

Check it out here → The Paleo Recipe Book

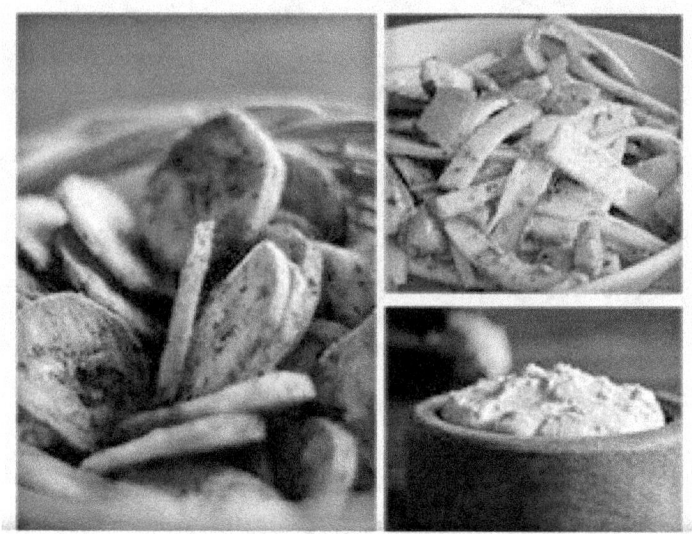
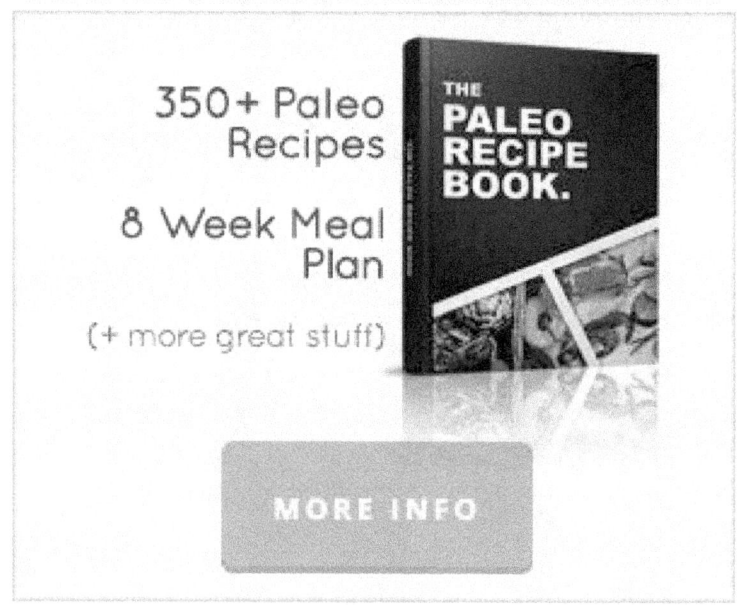

CONCLUSION

Thank you again for downloading this book!

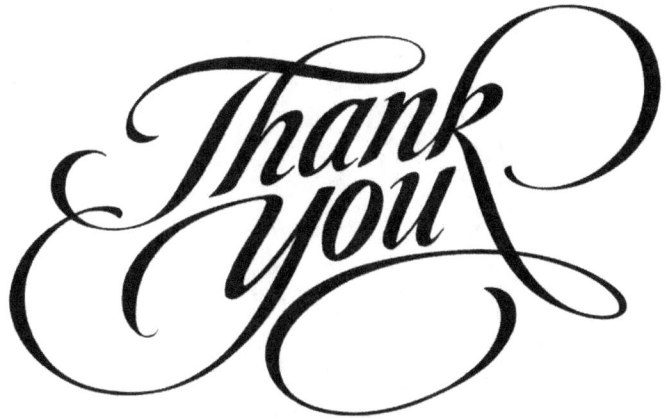

If you enjoyed this book, then I'd like to ask you for a favor, would you be kind enough to leave a review for this book on Amazon? It'd be greatly appreciated!

Help us better serve you by sending questions or comments to greatreadspublishing@gmail.com - Thank you!